Let's Get to the Point about Acupuncture!

Carolyn Provencher, R.Ac

Let's Get to the Point about Acupuncture!

Carolyn Provencher, R.Ac

Printed in the United States by Createspace
ISBN: 1539159493
ISBN -13: 978-1539159490

www.carolynprovencher.com

About the Author

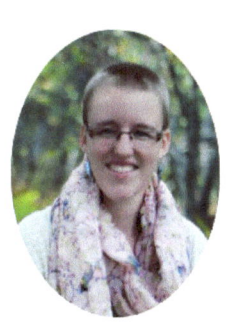

Carolyn Provencher, R.Ac holds a Masters of Science in Acupuncture from Southwest Acupuncture College in Boulder, CO. As an acupuncturist in the beautiful Upper Peninsula of Michigan, Carolyn specializes in working with people struggling with emotional distress and chronic illnesses. She is also author of *A Journal for your Acupuncture Journey* and co-author of the book *Tao Meets Now: A Clinical Manual of integrating 5 Element Acupuncture with Traditional Chinese Medicine* with Abbye Silverstein. When she is not in her clinic, Carolyn can most often be found exploring the wildernesses around her or on the dance floor with her husband. Find out more about Carolyn on her website **www.carolynprovencher.com**.

One question I am frequently asked as an acupuncturist is **"*How does acupuncture work?*"** Unfortunately, there is no easy way to explain it. Most of us are more comfortable with modern medicine and its connection to scientific methodology and straight forward answers to our issues. Acupuncture and Chinese Medicine, however, are based on Taoist Philosophy, where often answers are more poetic and less exact. Even the Chinese language is written as a series of characters that represent ideas. Each character is a picture and often includes the etiology of the concept, which can lead to an even deeper meaning of the word. For instance the character for Qi *(pronounced "chee")*:

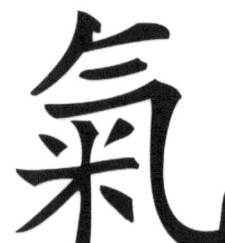

Qi is one of the most basic concepts in Chinese Medicine, however it does not translate nicely into English. Some texts translate it as "Vital Energy" that flows through the body, but even that explanation doesn't really embody the full concept of the term. Everything in life has Qi; it is the essence of life in all things. The character is a simplified image of steam rising from a grain of rice. The steam is what gives rice life and the ability to nourish our bodies. In a sense of eastern philosophy and poetry - that is what Qi is.

If you close your eyes and imagine that steam, can you feel it? What does that mean for you? Can you sense its energy?

Taoism is a way of looking at the world around us and relating that directly (and indirectly) to the world within us. Have you ever seen the "Yin-Yang" Symbol *(Yang rhymes with "Song")*? Have you ever wondered what it means? It represents one of the most basic principles in Chinese Medicine. Everything in life can be broken down into Yin and Yang, including all dis-ease within the body. The two concepts of yin and yang are independent of one another, but are also reliant on each other. Yin symbolizes the darkness, the winter, the stillness, the denseness, and the heaviness in life. Yang, on the other hand, represents the light, the summer, the floating, and the active. I like to think of Yin as the troll under the bridge, dark and rough on the edges; while Yang is the brightly colored songbird flying gracefully on the breeze. The goal of health is to keep both Yin & Yang in harmony throughout the body.

Our world is never entirely Yin or Yang, but rather constantly cycling through the phases of each. Through each day we watch as the darkness of midnight (most Yin) seamlessly moves into dawn, into noon (most Yang), into dusk, and back into midnight. Throughout the year we see winter (most Yin) transition into spring, into summer (most Yang), into autumn, and back to winter. It is a constant cycle that we can rely on and see day after day and year after year.

When Yin and Yang are broken down further, there are 5 distinct phases to this cycle: Water, Wood, Fire, Earth, and Metal. These are seen as the Five Elements, all acting upon and affecting

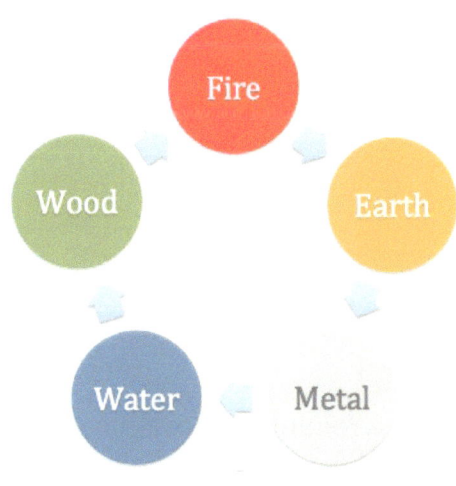

each other. In our bodies each of these Elements have a specific job, similar to the workings of a kingdom. Within the 5 Elements there are 12 Officials (2 Officials per Element, except Fire which holds 4 Officials). Each Official corresponds to an organ[1] in the body. I typically refer specifically to the individual Elements, but the Officials do shed light on the nuances of each Element. [See diagram on next page]

When all Five Elements, and consequently 12 Officials, are in balance, Yin and Yang are also in harmony, which is the definition of "health." Unfortunately life happens. Emotions, lifestyle choices, trauma, and injury can all affect certain Elements, which will in turn affect how the system as a whole functions. Acupuncture and Chinese Medicine can help bring these Elements, Yin and Yang back into balance.

Using needles, moxibustion, essential oils, flower essences, and bodywork techniques we can help guide your body back into its own balance. These techniques do not work overnight, but as we address each Element, you will start to feel better. The rest of this book goes into greater detail about each of these Elements and how it may be affecting your body.

---

[1] Just a reminder, that although these organs have been translated to share the name of an organ in modern science, it does not mean that the functions are considered to be exactly the same.

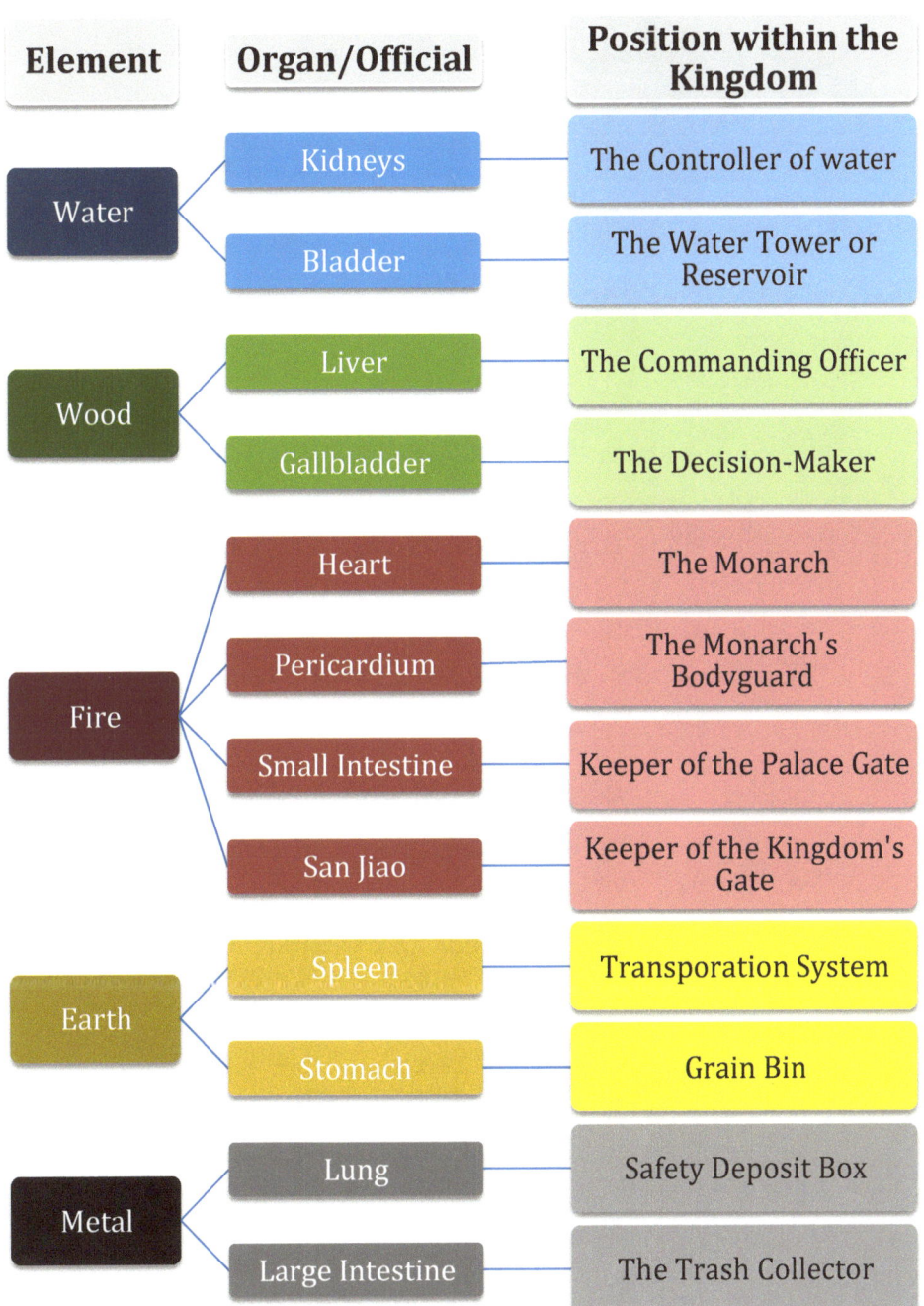

Element	Organ/Official	Position within the Kingdom
Water	Kidneys	The Controller of water
	Bladder	The Water Tower or Reservoir
Wood	Liver	The Commanding Officer
	Gallbladder	The Decision-Maker
Fire	Heart	The Monarch
	Pericardium	The Monarch's Bodyguard
	Small Intestine	Keeper of the Palace Gate
	San Jiao	Keeper of the Kingdom's Gate
Earth	Spleen	Transporation System
	Stomach	Grain Bin
Metal	Lung	Safety Deposit Box
	Large Intestine	The Trash Collector

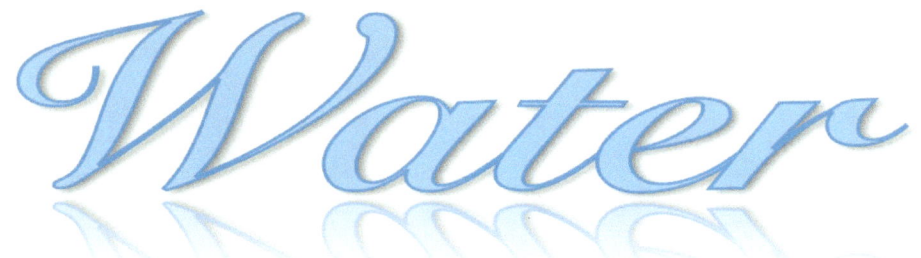

*W*ater holds its place in the cycle as the time between the end and the beginning. It is seen in the stillness of night and in the depths of winter. After death, the particles of a plant fall back into the ground where they become the soil, nutrients, and protection for new life to sprout and flourish.

Have you ever had a daily ritual, an idea, or even a friendship that you realized was no longer working for you? As those pieces of yourself began to disintegrate, the knowledge and wisdom you gained from those experiences became the nutrients and soil for a new seed to form. This new seed often needs time before it is ready to be seen or born; this gestation time is the Water Phase. It can be a time of chaos and unknowns. How does it feel?

When we start looking at the internal kingdom, the Water Element includes the Kidney and the Bladder. Similar to modern medicine, in the traditional texts both of these organs are associated with 'water' function in the body. As the kingdom's Officials, the Bladder's job is to store water, like a town's water tower. The Kidney uses that water and controls water usage within the kingdom.

As you can imagine, Water imbalances can arise as urinary imbalances, chronic dry cough, dry skin, and so on. More than that, the Water Element also overlaps with some parts of the endocrine system (specifically with the adrenal function in the body) and reproductive system.

The Water Element also includes a substance called *jing*. Jing is an essence that indicates longevity. It includes our ancestral history (DNA). Jing cannot be replaced, and is slowly used up as we grow older.

Overwork, chronic illness, addictive behaviors, and excessive fear can weaken the Water and use up jing more quickly. Symptoms can include depression, chronic fatigue, sexual imbalance, forgetfulness, urinary distress, bone disease, and hormonal imbalance. These symptoms are influenced not only by the Water Element, but also by the other four elements within the system.

Although acupuncture can't re-create jing for the body, it can help to balance the Water Element. By helping the Bladder to hold water more efficiently and helping the Kidney more effectively use this water, acupuncture can help your body metabolize and rest more effectively.

Wood

The Wood emerges from the Yin of darkness with a spark of Yang. With this spark of light the seed of Water splits open and drives us forward through life, allowing us to grow and develop.

As form begins to emerge from the chaos of the unknown, your own seed is able to sprout and grow into a beautiful reaching tree. Each branch stretching and reaching based on the potential of that small seed. How does it feel to stand tall and actively reach toward your dreams? How does it feel to make each decision based on that wisdom of deep inner knowing?

Looking a little deeper into the kingdom of our bodies, the Wood Element includes the Liver and Gallbladder Officials. If the Heart is the Emperor (we will get to that next), The Liver is the Commanding Officer, bringing the Heart's wishes into bodily form. Specifically, the Liver commands Xue, or as it often gets translated, Blood.

Xue includes blood, but it also includes Qi, hormones, and nutrients. Xue helps nourish bones, tendons, and the brain. The Liver's job is to ensure that Qi and Xue move smoothly and easily through the body to minimize pain and discomfort. The Commanding Officer's sidekick is the Gallbladder Official. His/her role is to make sure all the details are in order so that the Liver can effectively carry out the Emperor's orders.

When it comes to the Wood Element, we are most familiar with hardwood trees that stand tall and strong. This is only one aspect of the Wood Element. A healthy Wood Element also allows for flexibility in the wind and the waves like bamboo – strong and flexible. A healthy tree will help move the Xue, or blood, throughout the body, bringing nourishment to all of the limbs and systems.

However, emotional stress and lifestyle choices can cause havoc for this system. Irregular and/or painful periods, cold hands and feet, irritability, eye issues, tendon injuries, and tenderness in the chest and abdomen are all symptoms of Wood disharmonies.

Acupuncture is wonderful for helping to balance the Wood Element and assist it in directing Xue effectively throughout the body. When this happens, freedom of movement increases and stress decreases.

FIRE

The Fire Phase is the phase of most Yang – it is the guiding light at the end of the tunnel. As we move through the cycle, Fire can be seen in the warm sunshine of summer. The fire element is expressed when an individual discovers *"who I am"* or a plant shows its true colors.

As the stems and branches begin to unfurl from your once small seed, this now full and reaching tree can mature and identify itself and its place in the world. As the tree begins to flower, it is like dreams and desires coming to the light – they are identifiable and reachable. Take a moment to feel the warmth of love and passion that your soul has to offer during this time of understanding.

When in balance, the Fire Element allows us to feel love, passion, and joy. But it is easy for the Fire to blow out of proportion with all of that Yang energy flaming upwards. This can lead to sleep disturbances, anxiety, inability to focus, high blood pressure, ulcers, and digestive issues.

The ancient Chinese included four Officials in the Fire system. The Heart is considered the monarch or overseer of all of the other Officials. In order to protect the body's monarch, three other Officials have been employed:

- Pericardium – The Monarch's Bodyguard
- Small Intestine – Keeper of the Palace Gate
- San Jiao (Triple Warmer) – Keeper of the Kingdom's Gate

We are all familiar with the heart organ; it keeps us alive with its very steady and reliable *"lub-dub."* Around this monarchal organ is the protective sack of the pericardium allowing only the most sacred and pure to penetrate and reach the heart, ultimately becoming part of our being.

Both modern medicine and Chinese methodology agree that the small intestine is where 90% of nutrient absorption happens – constantly sorting between what is pure and beneficial to our body and what is impure. Like the palace's gatekeeper deciding who is can enter, getting one step closer to the emperor, and who needs to keep their distance.

The San Jiao (or Triple Warmer) is a concept rather than an organ. The job of the San Jiao often correlates with the thyroid and endocrine systems. It helps regulate the temperature and fluids in the body. Temperature imbalances, edema, and unexplained weight gain can often be addressed through the means of the San Jiao.

Acupuncture can help regulate the Fire Element – either firing up or calming down the flame. Although we can sometimes get immediate short-term results, these types of issues often take a while to address the root – we want to work with all the guards and protectors of the heart before working with the emperor, which is required for long-term health and well-being.

Earth

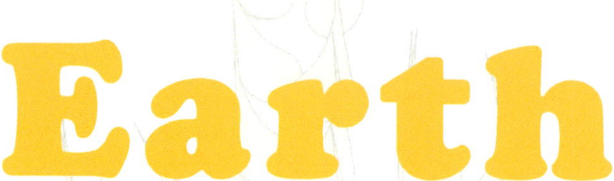

At the very end of summer, but before the fall, there is a slight change in the weather. The air starts to feel a little heavier and the bright and brilliant flowers begin to bear fruit. The harvest season has begun.

After we have isolated and identified our heart's desires, they begin to bear fruit – an offering to share. As we sing the song of our heart, we are given the opportunity to share our passions with those around us. In your own ecosystem, the sweet fruit and bounty is a gift for you. It comes in abundance. Soon the fruit will begin to grow heavy, over ripen, and rot. Take a moment to ground yourself and thank the Earth for all it has provided you in stability, loyalty, and nourishment.

Within our own internal kingdom, the Earth includes the Stomach and Spleen organs, which are considered the primary digestive tract. The Stomach is considered the grain bin for the kingdom, storing and ripening the food before the rest of the system uses it. The Spleen's job is to transport the fuel to where it is most needed. When in balance the Earth helps the body's digestive system, but also relates to mental clarity, focus, and muscular health.

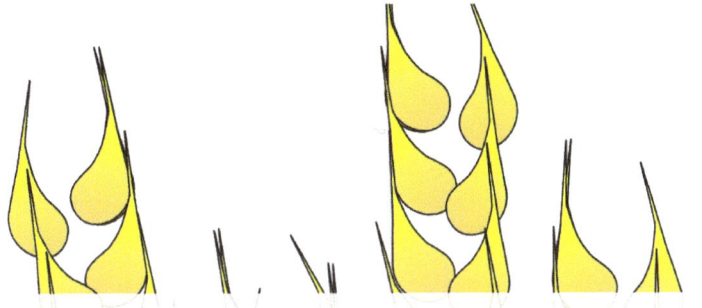

Therefore, imbalances in the Earth system can present as attention deficient disorder, eating disorders, and other forms of self-harm. On a more physical level, digestive upsets including nausea, vomiting, constipation, and diarrhea are also strongly influenced by the Earth Element. Modern medicine is also seeing some of these connections – there are multiple new studies coming out looking at how gut health can help with brain function and focus potential.

The Earth holds the space for the other Four Elements – oceans, trees, flowers, and mountains. It cares for these Elements and provides them everything they need to survive. It also establishes the boundaries that each needs, just as a mother does for each of her children. And just like that mother, the Earth Element is the caretaker of the body, providing nourishment and support for the whole self – body, mind, and spirit.

Acupuncture can also help nourish our Earth by supporting the Earth itself and by helping to dial back the other elements and remind them to respect Earth's boundaries. Good eating habits are an important part of the Earth's health. It isn't so much what you eat, but how you eat. Mindful eating gives space, time, and connection in order to focus on nourishing our self and our body each day.

Metal

Metal materializes when the fruit gives way and begins to decompose back into the soil, the leaves begin to turn, and the Earth prepares for the darkness and stillness ahead. It is seen at dusk as the sun sinks under the horizon.

As your own body prepares for the upcoming transition from the Metal to the Water Element, how does it feel to watch the leaves of your life change colors and transform before seamlessly falling to the ground? What does it feel like to let go and surrender to this transformation?

The Metal Element brings a rhythmic order to the mystery of life and death. Metal distinguishes only between black and white, life and death, holding on and letting go. However, when in balance with the other elements, it also allows us to appreciate the beauty and preciousness that life makes available to us. And within that we are able to feel the sensations of the world around us that inspire to connect with the universe as a whole.

The Metal system relates to the Lungs and Large Intestine Officials.

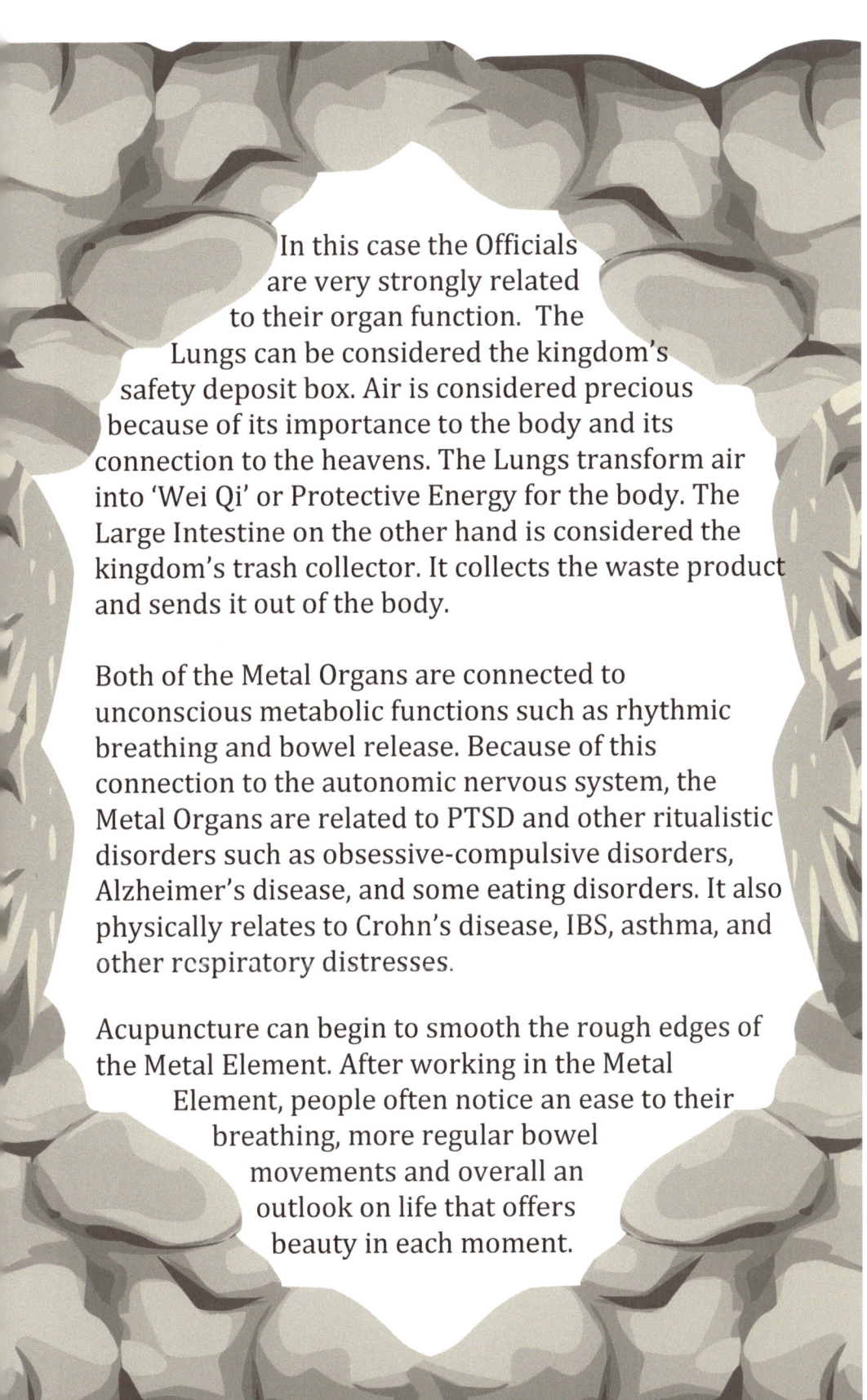

In this case the Officials are very strongly related to their organ function. The Lungs can be considered the kingdom's safety deposit box. Air is considered precious because of its importance to the body and its connection to the heavens. The Lungs transform air into 'Wei Qi' or Protective Energy for the body. The Large Intestine on the other hand is considered the kingdom's trash collector. It collects the waste product and sends it out of the body.

Both of the Metal Organs are connected to unconscious metabolic functions such as rhythmic breathing and bowel release. Because of this connection to the autonomic nervous system, the Metal Organs are related to PTSD and other ritualistic disorders such as obsessive-compulsive disorders, Alzheimer's disease, and some eating disorders. It also physically relates to Crohn's disease, IBS, asthma, and other respiratory distresses.

Acupuncture can begin to smooth the rough edges of the Metal Element. After working in the Metal Element, people often notice an ease to their breathing, more regular bowel movements and overall an outlook on life that offers beauty in each moment.

Date: _____

Any significant events or goals for your day?

How is your energy level today?

(None) 1   2   3   4   5   6   7   8   9   10 (Excess)

Did you have **acupuncture** or **other therapy** today?   Yes   No
Did you add or **change any medications** today?   Yes   No

How are you feeling today? Mark any that you connect with.

Accepted	Amazed	Amused	Annoyed	Anxious
Balanced	Bold	Calm	Comfortable	Confident
Depressed	Disgusted	Doubtful	Ecstatic	Energized
Enraged	Enthusiastic	Euphoric	Excited	Expansive
Fearful	Focused	Frisky	Grounded	Guilty
Inspired	Irritated	Joyous	Letdown	Liberated
Lifeless	Lonely	Lost	Loved	Loving
Off-Kilter	Overwhelm	Paranoid	Passionate	Peaceful
Playful	Radiant	Rejected	Relaxed	Resentful
Reserved	Revengeful	Satisfied	Self-Hating	Spunky
Stressed	Supported	Tense	Thankful	Trapped

Others: _____

How are you physical feeling today?

Pain: _____

Digestion/Bowel: _____

Appetite: _____

Menstruation: _____

Exercise: _____

Other: _____

Take a moment to process your day. What made today different or special? Do this in your own way: write, paint, draw, color, photos, collage, or anything else you can think of.

"Forgiving those who hurt us is the key to personal peace" ~G. Weatherly

Date: _____

Any significant events or goals for your day?

How is your energy level today?

(None) 1   2   3   4   5   6   7   8   9   10 (Excess)

Did you have **acupuncture** or **other therapy** today?   Yes   No
Did you add or **change any medications** today?   Yes   No

How are you feeling today? Mark any that you connect with.

Accepted	Amazed	Amused	Annoyed	Anxious
Balanced	Bold	Calm	Comfortable	Confident
Depressed	Disgusted	Doubtful	Ecstatic	Energized
Enraged	Enthusiastic	Euphoric	Excited	Expansive
Fearful	Focused	Frisky	Grounded	Guilty
Inspired	Irritated	Joyous	Letdown	Liberated
Lifeless	Lonely	Lost	Loved	Loving
Off-Kilter	Overwhelm	Paranoid	Passionate	Peaceful
Playful	Radiant	Rejected	Relaxed	Resentful
Reserved	Revengeful	Satisfied	Self-Hating	Spunky
Ungrounded	Unworthy	Useless	Withdrawn	Worried

Others: _____

How are you physical feeling today?

Pain: _____

Digestion/Bowel: _____

Appetite: _____

Menstruation: _____

Exercise: _____

Other: _____

Take a moment to process your day? What made today different or special? Do this in your own way: write, paint, draw, color, photos, collage, or anything else you can think of.

Date: _____

Any significant events or goals for your day?

How is your energy level today?

(None) 1   2   3   4   5   6   7   8   9   10 (Excess)

Did you have **acupuncture** or **other therapy** today?   Yes   No
Did you add or **change any medications** today?   Yes   No

How are you feeling today? Mark any that you connect with.

Accepted	Amazed	Amused	Annoyed	Anxious
Balanced	Bold	Calm	Comfortable	Confident
Depressed	Disgusted	Doubtful	Ecstatic	Energized
Enraged	Enthusiastic	Euphoric	Excited	Expansive
Fearful	Focused	Frisky	Grounded	Guilty
Inspired	Irritated	Joyous	Letdown	Liberated
Lifeless	Lonely	Lost	Loved	Loving
Off-Kilter	Overwhelm	Paranoid	Passionate	Peaceful
Playful	Radiant	Rejected	Relaxed	Resentful
Stressed	Supported	Tense	Thankful	Trapped
Ungrounded	Unworthy	Useless	Withdrawn	Worried

Others: _____

How are you physical feeling today?

Pain: _____

Digestion/Bowel: _____

Appetite: _____

Menstruation: _____

Exercise: _____

Other: _____

Take a moment to process your day. What made today different or special? Do this in your own way: write, paint, draw, color, photos, collage, or anything else you can think of.

Do you what to find out more?

Carolyn Provencher Acupuncture

906-458-2565

www.carolynprovencher.com